INDIAN COOKBOOK 2021

TASTY INDIAN RECIPES MADE EASY AND FAST

AGNI BAKSHI

Table of Contents

Instant Dosa 12
    Ingredients 12
    Method 13
Sweet Potato Roll 14
    Ingredients 14
    Method 14
Potato Pancake 15
    Ingredients 15
    Method 16
Murgh Malai Kebab 17
    Ingredients 17
    Method 18
Keema Puffs 19
    Ingredients 19
    Method 20
Egg Pakoda 21
    Ingredients 21
    Method 21
Egg Dosa 22
    Ingredients 22
    Method 23
Khasta Kachori 24
    Ingredients 24

- Method 25
- Mixed Legume Dhokla 26
  - Ingredients 26
  - Method 27
- Frankie 28
  - Ingredients 28
  - Method 29
- Besan & Cheese Delight 30
  - Ingredients 30
  - For the besan mix: 30
  - Method 31
- Chilli Idli 32
  - Ingredients 32
  - Method 32
- Spinach Canapé 33
  - Ingredients 33
  - Method 34
- Paushtik Chaat 35
  - Ingredients 35
  - Method 36
- Cabbage Roll 37
  - Ingredients 37
  - Method 38
- Tomato Bread 39
  - Ingredients 39
  - Method 39
- Corn & Cheese Balls 40

- Ingredients 40
- Method 40

Corn Flakes Chivda 41
- Ingredients 41
- Method 42

Nut Roll 43
- Ingredients 43
- Method 44

Cabbage Rolls with Mince 45
- Ingredients 45
- Method 46

Pav Bhaji 47
- Ingredients 47
- Method 48

Soy Cutlet 49
- Ingredients 49
- Method 49

Corn Bhel 51
- Ingredients 51
- Method 51

Methi Gota 52
- Ingredients 52
- Method 53

Idli 54
- Ingredients 54
- Method 54

Idli Plus 55

- Ingredients 55
  - Method 56
- Masala Sandwich 57
  - Ingredients 57
  - Method 58
- Mint Kebab 59
  - Ingredients 59
  - Method 59
- Vegetable Sevia Upma 60
  - Ingredients 60
  - Method 61
- Bhel 62
  - Ingredients 62
  - Method 62
- Sabudana Khichdi 63
  - Ingredients 63
  - Method 64
- Simple Dhokla 65
  - Ingredients 65
  - Method 66
- Jaldi Potato 67
  - Ingredients 67
  - Method 67
- Orange Dhokla 68
  - Ingredients 68
  - Method 69
- Cabbage Muthia 70

- Ingredients 70
  - Method 71
- Rava Dhokla 72
  - Ingredients 72
  - Method 72
- Chapatti Upma 73
  - Ingredients 73
  - Method 74
- Mung Dhokla 75
  - Ingredients 75
  - Method 75
- Mughlai Meat Cutlet 76
  - Ingredients 76
  - Method 77
- Masala Vada 78
  - Ingredients 78
  - Method 78
- Cabbage Chivda 79
  - Ingredients 79
  - Method 80
- Bread Besan Bhajji 81
  - Ingredients 81
  - Method 81
- Methi Seekh Kebab 82
  - Ingredients 82
  - Method 82
- Jhinga Hariyali 83

Ingredients	83
Method	84
Methi Adai	**85**
Ingredients	85
Method	86
Peas Chaat	**87**
Ingredients	87
Method	87
Shingada	**88**
Ingredients	88
For the pastry:	88
Method	89
Onion Bhajia	**90**
Ingredients	90
Method	90
Bagani Murgh	**91**
Ingredients	91
For the marinade:	91
Method	92
Potato Tikki	**93**
Ingredients	93
Method	94
Batata Vada	**95**
Ingredients	95
Method	96
Mini Chicken Kebab	**97**
Ingredients	97

- Method 97
- Lentil Rissole 98
  - Ingredients 98
  - Method 99
- Nutritious Poha 100
  - Ingredients 100
  - Method 100
- Beans Usal 101
  - Ingredients 101
  - Method 102
- Bread Chutney Pakoda 103
  - Ingredients 103
  - Method 103
- Methi Khakra Delight 104
  - Ingredients 104
  - Method 104
- Green Cutlet 105
  - Ingredients 105
  - Method 106
- Handvo 107
  - Ingredients 107
  - Method 108
- Ghugra 109
  - Ingredients 109
  - Method 109
- Banana Kebab 111
  - Ingredients 111

Method..111

Instant Dosa

(Instant Rice Crêpe)

Makes 10-12

Ingredients

85g/3oz rice flour

45g/1½oz wholemeal flour

45g/1½oz plain white flour

25g/scant 1oz semolina

60g/2oz besan*

1 tsp ground cumin

4 green chillies, finely chopped

2 tbsp sour cream

Salt to taste

120ml/4fl oz refined vegetable oil

Method

- Mix together all the ingredients, except the oil, with enough water to make a thick batter of a pouring consistency.

- Heat a frying pan and pour a tsp of the oil in it. Pour 2 tbsp of the batter and spread with the back of a spoon to make a crêpe.

- Cook on a low heat till the underside is brown. Flip and repeat.

- Remove carefully with a spatula. Repeat for the remaining batter.

- Serve hot with any chutney.

Sweet Potato Roll

Makes 15-20

Ingredients

4 large sweet potatoes, steamed and mashed

175g/6oz rice flour

4 tbsp honey

20 cashew nuts, lightly roasted and chopped

20 raisins

Salt to taste

2 tsp sesame seeds

Ghee for deep frying

Method

- Mix together all the ingredients, except the ghee and the sesame seeds.

- Make walnut-sized balls and roll in the sesame seeds to coat.

- Heat the ghee in a frying pan. Deep fry the balls on a medium heat till golden brown. Serve hot.

Potato Pancake

Makes 30

Ingredients

6 large potatoes, 3 grated plus 3 boiled and mashed

2 eggs

2 tbsp plain white flour

½ tsp freshly ground black pepper

1 small onion, finely chopped

120ml /4fl oz milk

60ml/2fl oz refined vegetable oil

1 tsp salt

2 tbsp oil

Method

- Mix together all the ingredients, except the oil, to form a thick batter.

- Heat a flat pan and spread the oil on it. Drop 2-4 large spoonfuls of the batter and spread like a pancake.

- Cook each side on a medium heat for 3-4 minutes till the pancake is golden and crisp around the edges.

- Repeat for the remaining batter. Serve hot.

Murgh Malai Kebab

(Creamy Chicken Kebab)

Makes 25-30

Ingredients

1 tsp ginger paste

1 tsp garlic paste

2 green chillies

25g/scant 1oz coriander leaves, finely chopped

3 tbsp cream

1 tsp plain white flour

125g/4½oz Cheddar cheese, grated

1 tsp salt

500g/1lb 2oz boneless chicken, finely chopped

Method

- Mix together all the ingredients, except the chicken.

- Marinate the chicken pieces with the mixture for 4-6 hours.

- Arrange in an ovenproof dish and bake in an oven at 165ºC (325ºF, Gas Mark 4) for about 20-30 minutes, till the chicken turns light brown.

- Serve hot with mint chutney

Keema Puffs

(Mince-stuffed Savouries)

Makes 12

Ingredients

250g/9oz plain white flour

½ tbsp salt

½ tsp baking powder

1 tbsp ghee

100ml/3½fl oz water

2 tbsp refined vegetable oil

2 medium-sized onions, finely chopped

¾ tsp ginger paste

¾ tsp garlic paste

6 green chillies, finely chopped

1 large tomato, finely chopped

½ tsp turmeric

½ tsp chilli powder

1 tsp garam masala

125g/4½oz frozen peas

4 tbsp yoghurt

2 tbsp water

50g/1¾oz coriander leaves, finely chopped

500g/1lb 2oz chicken, minced

Method

- Sieve together the flour, salt and baking powder. Add the ghee and water. Knead to form a dough. Set aside for 30 minutes and knead once again. Set aside.

- Heat the oil in a saucepan. Add the onions, ginger paste, garlic paste and green chillies. Fry for 2 minutes on a medium heat.

- Add the tomato, turmeric, chilli powder, garam masala and some salt. Mix well and cook for 5 minutes, stirring frequently.

- Add the peas, yoghurt, water, coriander leaves and the minced chicken. Mix well. Cook for 15 minutes, stirring occasionally, till the mixture becomes dry. Set aside.

- Roll out the dough into one big disc. Cut into a square shape, then cut 12 small rectangles out of the square.

- Place the mince mixture in the centre of each rectangle and roll like a candy wrapper.

- Bake in an oven at 175ºC (350ºF, Gas Mark 4) for 10 minutes. Serve hot.

Egg Pakoda

(Fried Egg Snack)

Makes 20

Ingredients

3 eggs, whisked

3 bread slices, quartered

125g/4½oz Cheddar cheese, grated

1 onion, finely chopped

3 green chillies, finely chopped

1 tbsp coriander leaves chopped

½ tsp ground black pepper

½ tsp chilli powder

Salt to taste

Refined vegetable oil for deep frying

Method

- Mix together all the ingredients, except the oil.

- Heat the oil in a frying pan. Add spoonfuls of the mixture. Fry on a medium heat till golden brown.

- Drain on absorbent paper. Serve hot.

Egg Dosa

(Egg and Rice Crêpe)

Makes 12-14

Ingredients

150g/5½oz urad dhal*

100g/3½oz steamed rice

Salt to taste

4 eggs, whisked

Ground black pepper to taste

25g/scant 1oz onion, finely chopped

2 tbsp coriander leaves chopped

1 tbsp refined vegetable oil

1 tbsp butter

Method

- Soak the dhal and rice together for 4 hours. Add salt and grind to a thick batter. Let it ferment overnight.

- Grease and heat a flat pan. Spread 2 tbsp of the batter over it.

- Pour 3 tbsp of the egg over the batter. Sprinkle pepper, onion and coriander leaves. Pour some oil around the edges and cook for 2 minutes. Flip carefully and cook for 2 more minutes.

- Repeat for the rest of the batter. Place a knob of butter on each dosa and serve hot with coconut chutney

Khasta Kachori

(Spicy Fried Lentil Dumpling)

Makes 12-15

Ingredients

200g/7oz besan*

300g/10oz plain white flour

Salt to taste

200ml/7fl oz water

2 tbsp refined vegetable oil plus for deep frying

Pinch of asafoetida

225g/8oz mung dhal*, soaked for an hour and drained

1 tsp turmeric

1 tsp ground coriander

4 tsp fennel seeds

2-3 cloves

1 tbsp coriander leaves, finely chopped

3 green chillies, finely chopped

2.5cm/1in root ginger, finely chopped

1 tbsp mint leaves, finely chopped

¼ tsp chilli powder

1 tsp amchoor*

Method

- Knead the besan, flour and some salt with enough water into a stiff dough. Set aside.

- Heat the oil in a saucepan. Add the asafoetida and let it splutter for 15 seconds. Add the dhal and fry for 5 minutes on a medium heat, stirring continuously.

- Add the turmeric, ground coriander, fennel seeds, cloves, coriander leaves, green chillies, ginger, mint leaves, chilli powder and amchoor. Mix well and cook for 10-12 minutes. Set aside.

- Divide the dough into lemon-sized balls. Flatten them and roll out into small discs, 12.5cm/5in in diameter.

- Place a spoonful of the dhal mixture in the centre of each disc. Seal like a pouch and flatten into puris. Set aside.

- Heat the oil in a saucepan. Deep fry the puris till they puff up.

- Serve hot with green coconut chutney

Mixed Legume Dhokla

(Steamed Mixed Legume Cake)

Makes 20

Ingredients

125g/4½oz whole mung beans*

125g/4½oz kaala chana*

60g/2oz Turkish gram

50g/1¾oz dry green peas

75g/2½oz urad beans*

2 tsp green chillies

Salt to taste

Method

- Soak together the mung beans, kaala chana, Turkish gram and dry green peas. Soak the urad beans separately. Set aside for 6 hours.

- Grind all the soaked ingredients together to make a thick batter. Ferment for 6 hours.

- Add the green chillies and salt. Mix well and pour into a 20cm/8in round cake tin and steam for 10 minutes.

- Cut into diamond shapes. Serve with mint chutney

Frankie

Makes 10-12

Ingredients

1 tsp chaat masala*

½ tsp garam masala

½ tsp ground cumin

4 large potatoes, boiled and mashed

Salt to taste

10-12 chapattis

Refined vegetable oil for greasing

2-3 green chillies, chopped finely and soaked in some white vinegar

2 tbsp coriander leaves, finely chopped

1 onion, finely chopped

Method

- Mix together the chaat masala, garam masala, ground cumin, potatoes and salt. Knead well and set aside.

- Heat a frying pan and place a chapatti on it.

- Spread a little oil on the chapatti and flip it to fry one side. Repeat for the other side.

- Spread a layer of the potato mixture evenly on the hot chapatti.

- Sprinkle a few green chillies, coriander leaves and onion.

- Roll up the chapatti so that the potato mixture is inside.

- Dry roast the roll on the frying pan till golden brown and serve hot.

Besan & Cheese Delight

Makes 25

Ingredients

2 eggs

250g/9oz Cheddar cheese, grated

1 tsp ground black pepper

1 tsp ground mustard

½ tsp chilli powder

60ml/2fl oz refined vegetable oil

For the besan mix:

50g/1¾oz semolina, dry roasted

375g/13oz besan*

200g/7oz cabbage, grated

1 tsp ginger paste

1 tsp garlic paste

Pinch of baking powder

Salt to taste

Method

- Whisk 1 egg thoroughly. Add the Cheddar cheese, pepper, ground mustard and chilli powder. Mix well and set aside.

- Mix the besan mix ingredients together. Transfer to a 20cm/8in round cake tin and steam for 20 minutes. When cooled, cut into 25 pieces and spread the egg-cheese mixture over each.

- Heat the oil in a saucepan. Deep fry the pieces on a medium heat till golden brown. Serve hot with green coconut chutney

Chilli Idli

Serves 4

Ingredients

3 tbsp refined vegetable oil

1 tsp mustard seeds

1 small onion, sliced

½ tsp garam masala

1 tbsp ketchup

4 idlis chopped

Salt to taste

2 tbsp coriander leaves

Method

- Heat the oil in a saucepan. Add the mustard seeds. Let them splutter for 15 seconds.

- Add all the remaining ingredients, except the coriander leaves. Mix well.

- Cook on a medium heat for 4-5 minutes, tossing gently. Garnish with the coriander leaves. Serve hot.

Spinach Canapé

Makes 10

Ingredients

2 tbsp butter

10 bread slices, quartered

2 tbsp ghee

1 onion, finely chopped

300g/10oz spinach, finely chopped

Salt to taste

125g/4½oz goat's cheese, drained

4 tbsp Cheddar cheese, grated

Method

- Butter both sides of the bread pieces and bake in a preheated oven at 200ºC (400ºF, Gas Mark 6) for 7 minutes. Set aside.

- Heat the ghee in a saucepan. Fry the onion till brown. Add the spinach and salt. Cook for 5 minutes. Add the goat's cheese and mix well.

- Spread the spinach mixture on the toasted bread pieces. Sprinkle some grated Cheddar cheese on top and bake in an oven at 130°C (250°F, Gas Mark ½) till the cheese melts. Serve hot.

Paushtik Chaat

(Healthy Snack)

Serves 4

Ingredients

3 tsp refined vegetable oil

½ tsp cumin seeds

2.5cm/1in root ginger, crushed

1 small potato, boiled and chopped

1 tsp garam masala

Salt to taste

Ground black pepper to taste

250g/9oz mung beans, cooked

300g/10oz canned kidney beans

300g/10oz canned chickpeas

10g/¼oz coriander leaves, chopped

1 tsp lemon juice

Method

- Heat the oil in a saucepan. Add the cumin seeds. Let them splutter for 15 seconds.
- Add the ginger, potato, garam masala, salt and pepper. Sauté on a medium heat for 3 minutes. Add the mung beans, kidney beans and chickpeas. Cook on a medium heat for 8 minutes.
- Garnish with the coriander leaves and lemon juice. Serve chilled.

Cabbage Roll

Serves 4

Ingredients

1 tbsp plain white flour

3 tbsp water

Salt to taste

2 tbsp refined vegetable oil plus for deep frying

1 tsp cumin seeds

100g/3½oz frozen, mixed vegetables

1 tbsp single cream

2 tbsp paneer*

¼ tsp turmeric

1 tsp chilli powder

1 tsp ground coriander

1 tsp ground cumin

8 big cabbage leaves, soaked in hot water for 2-3 minutes and drained

Method

- Mix the flour, water and salt to form a thick paste. Set aside.
- Heat the oil in a saucepan. Add the cumin seeds and let them splutter for 15 seconds. Add all the remaining ingredients, except the cabbage leaves. Cook on a medium heat for 2-3 minutes, stirring frequently.
- Place spoonfuls of this mixture in the centre of each cabbage leaf. Fold the leaves up and seal the ends with the flour paste.
- Heat the oil in a frying pan. Dip the cabbage rolls in the flour paste and deep fry. Serve hot.

Tomato Bread

Makes 4

Ingredients

1½ tbsp refined vegetable oil

150g/5½oz tomato purée

3-4 curry leaves

2 green chillies, finely chopped

Salt to taste

2 large potatoes, boiled and sliced

6 bread slices, shredded

10g/¼oz coriander leaves, chopped

Method

- Heat the oil in a saucepan. Add the tomato purée, curry leaves, green chillies and salt. Cook for 5 minutes.
- Add the potatoes and the bread. Cook on a low heat for 5 minutes.
- Garnish with the coriander leaves. Serve hot.

Corn & Cheese Balls

Makes 8-10

Ingredients

200g/7oz sweet corn

250g/9oz Mozzarella cheese, grated

4 large potatoes, boiled and mashed

2 green chillies, finely chopped

2.5cm/1in root ginger, finely chopped

1 tbsp coriander leaves, chopped

1 tsp lemon juice

50g/1¾oz breadcrumbs

Salt to taste

Refined vegetable oil for deep frying

50g/1¾oz semolina

Method

- In a bowl, mix together all the ingredients, except the oil and the semolina. Divide into 8-10 balls.
- Heat the oil in a saucepan. Roll the balls in the semolina and deep fry on a medium heat till golden brown. Serve hot.

Corn Flakes Chivda

(Roasted Corn Flakes Snack)

Makes 500g/1lb 2oz

Ingredients

250g/9oz peanuts

150g/5½oz chana dhal*

100g/3½oz raisins

125g/4½oz cashew nuts

200g/7oz cornflakes

60ml/2fl oz refined vegetable oil

7 green chillies, slit

25 curry leaves

½ tsp turmeric

2 tsp sugar

Salt to taste

Method

- Dry roast the peanuts, chana dhal, raisins, cashew nuts and cornflakes till crisp. Set aside.
- Heat the oil in a saucepan. Add the green chillies, curry leaves and turmeric. Sauté on a medium heat for a minute.
- Add the sugar, salt and all the roasted ingredients. Stir-fry for 2-3 minutes.
- Cool and store in an airtight container for up to 8 days.

Nut Roll

Makes 20-25

Ingredients

140g/5oz plain white flour

240ml/8fl oz milk

1 tbsp butter

Salt to taste

Ground black pepper to taste

½ tbsp coriander leaves, finely chopped

3-4 tbsp Cheddar cheese, grated

¼ tsp nutmeg, grated

125g/4½oz cashew nuts, coarsely ground

125g/4½oz peanuts, coarsely ground

50g/1¾oz breadcrumbs

Refined vegetable oil for deep frying

Method

- Mix 85g/3oz flour with the milk in a saucepan. Add the butter and cook the mixture, stirring continuously, on a low heat till it is thick.
- Add the salt and pepper. Let the mixture cool for 20 minutes.
- Add the coriander leaves, Cheddar cheese, nutmeg, cashew nuts and peanuts. Mix thoroughly. Set aside.
- Sprinkle half the breadcrumbs on a tray.
- Drop teaspoonfuls of the flour mixture over the breadcrumbs and make rolls. Set aside.
- Mix the remaining flour with enough water to make a thin batter. Dip the rolls in the batter and roll them again in breadcrumbs.
- Heat the oil in a saucepan. Deep fry the rolls on a medium heat till light brown.
- Serve hot with ketchup or green coconut chutney

Cabbage Rolls with Mince

Makes 12

Ingredients

1 tbsp refined vegetable oil plus extra for frying

2 onions, finely chopped

2 tomatoes, finely chopped

½ tbsp ginger paste

½ tbsp garlic paste

2 green chillies, sliced

½ tsp turmeric

½ tsp chilli powder

¼ tsp ground black pepper

500g/1lb 2oz chicken, minced

200g/7oz frozen peas

2 small potatoes, diced

1 big carrot, diced

Salt to taste

25g/scant 1oz coriander leaves, finely chopped

12 large cabbage leaves, parboiled

2 eggs whisked

100g/3½oz breadcrumbs

Method

- Heat 1 tbsp oil in a saucepan. Fry the onions till translucent.
- Add the tomatoes, ginger paste, garlic paste, green chillies, turmeric, chilli powder and pepper. Mix well and fry for 2 minutes on a medium heat.
- Add the chicken mince, peas, potatoes, carrots, salt and coriander leaves. Simmer for 20-30 minutes, stirring occasionally. Cool the mixture for 20 minutes.
- Place spoonfulls of the mince mixture in a cabbage leaf and roll it. Repeat for the remaining leaves. Secure the rolls with a toothpick.
- Heat the oil in a saucepan. Dip the rolls in the egg, coat with the breadcrumbs and fry till golden brown.
- Drain and serve hot.

Pav Bhaji

(Spicy Vegetables with Bread)

Serves 4

Ingredients

2 large potatoes, boiled

200g/7oz frozen, mixed vegetables (green peppers, carrots, cauliflower and peas)

2 tbsp butter

1½ tsp garlic paste

2 large onions, grated

4 large tomatoes, chopped

250ml/8fl oz water

2 tsp pav bhaji masala*

1½ tsp chilli powder

¼ tsp turmeric

Juice of 1 lemon

Salt to taste

1 tbsp coriander leaves, chopped

Butter to roast

4 hamburger buns, slit into half

1 large onion, finely chopped

Small slices of lemon

Method

- Mash the vegetables well. Set aside.
- Heat the butter in a saucepan. Add the garlic paste and onions and fry till the onions turn brown. Add the tomatoes and fry, stirring occasionally, on a medium heat for 10 minutes.
- Add the mashed vegetables, water, pav bhaji masala, chilli powder, turmeric, lemon juice and salt. Simmer till the gravy is thick. Mash and cook for 3-4 minutes, stirring continuously. Sprinkle the coriander leaves and mix well. Set aside.
- Heat a flat pan. Spread some butter on it and roast the hamburger buns till crisp on both sides.
- Serve the vegetables mixture hot with the buns, with the onion and lemon slices on the side.

Soy Cutlet

Makes 10

Ingredients

300g/10oz mung dhal*, soaked for 4 hours

Salt to taste

400g/14oz soy granules, soaked in warm water for 15 minutes

1 large onion, finely chopped

2-3 green chillies, finely chopped

1 tsp amchoor*

1 tsp garam masala

2 tbsp coriander leaves, chopped

150g/5½oz paneer* or tofu, grated

Refined vegetable oil for deep frying

Method

- Do not drain the dhal. Add the salt and cook in a saucepan on a medium heat for 40 minutes. Set aside.
- Drain the soy granules. Mix with the dhal and grind into a thick paste.
- In a non-stick saucepan, mix this paste with all the remaining ingredients, except the oil. Cook on a low heat till dry.

- Divide the mixture into lemon-sized balls and shape into cutlets.
- Heat the oil in a saucepan. Fry the cutlets till golden brown.
- Serve hot with mint chutney

Corn Bhel

(Spicy Corn Snack)

Serves 4

Ingredients

200g/7oz boiled corn kernels

100g/3½oz spring onions, finely chopped

1 potato, boiled, peeled and finely chopped

1 tomato, finely chopped

1 cucumber, finely chopped

10g/¼oz coriander leaves, chopped

1 tsp chaat masala*

2 tsp lemon juice

1 tbsp mint chutney

Salt to taste

Method

- In a bowl, toss all the ingredients together to mix thoroughly.
- Serve immediately.

Methi Gota

(Fried Fenugreek Dumpling)

Makes 20

Ingredients

500g/1lb 2oz besan*

45g/1½oz wholemeal flour

125g/4½oz yoghurt

4 tbsp refined vegetable oil plus extra for frying

2 tsp bicarbonate of soda

50g/1¾oz fresh fenugreek leaves, finely chopped

50g/1¾oz coriander leaves, finely chopped

1 ripe banana, peeled and mashed

1 tbsp coriander seeds

10-15 black peppercorns

2 green chillies

½ tsp ginger paste

½ tsp garam masala

Pinch of asafoetida

1 tsp chilli powder

Salt to taste

Method

- Mix the besan, flour and yoghurt together.
- Add 2 tbsp oil and the bicarbonate of soda. Set aside to ferment for 2-3 hours.
- Add all the remaining ingredients, except the oil. Mix well to make a thick batter.
- Heat 2 tbsp oil and add to the batter. Mix well and set aside for 5 minutes.
- Heat the remaining oil in a saucepan. Drop small spoonfuls of the batter into the oil and fry till golden brown.
- Drain on absorbent paper. Serve hot.

Idli

(Steamed Rice Cake)

Serves 4

Ingredients

500g/1lb 2oz rice, soaked overnight

300g/10oz urad dhal*, soaked overnight

1 tbsp salt

Pinch of bicarbonate of soda

Refined vegetable oil for greasing

Method

- Drain the rice and the dhal and grind together.
- Add the salt and bicarbonate of soda. Set aside for 8-9 hours to ferment.
- Grease cupcake moulds. Pour the rice-dhal mixture into them such that each is half-full. Steam for 10-12 minutes.
- Scoop the idlis out. Serve hot with coconut chutney

Idli Plus

(Steamed Rice Cake with Seasoning)

Serves 6

Ingredients

500g/1lb 2oz rice, soaked overnight

300g/10oz urad dhal*, soaked overnight

1 tbsp salt

¼ tsp turmeric

1 tbsp caster sugar

Salt to taste

1 tbsp refined vegetable oil

½ tsp cumin seeds

½ tsp mustard seeds

Method

- Drain the rice and the dhal and grind together.
- Add the salt and set aside for 8-9 hours to ferment.
- Add the turmeric, sugar and salt. Mix well and set aside.
- Heat the oil in a saucepan. Add the cumin and mustard seeds. Let them splutter for 15 seconds.
- Add the rice-dhal mixture. Cover with a lid and simmer for 10 minutes.
- Uncover and flip the mixture. Cover again and simmer for 5 minutes.
- Pierce the idli with a fork. If the fork comes out clean, the idli is done.
- Cut into pieces and serve hot with coconut chutney

Masala Sandwich

Makes 6

Ingredients

2 tsp refined vegetable oil

1 small onion, finely chopped

¼ tsp turmeric

1 large tomato, finely chopped

1 large potato, boiled and mashed

1 tbsp boiled peas

1 tsp chaat masala*

Salt to taste

10g/¼oz coriander leaves, chopped

50g/1¾oz butter

12 bread slices

Method

- Heat the oil in a saucepan. Add the onion and fry till translucent.
- Add the turmeric and tomato. Stir-fry on a medium heat for 2-3 minutes.
- Add the potato, peas, chaat masala, salt and coriander leaves. Mix well and cook for a minute on a low heat. Set aside.
- Butter the bread slices. Place a layer of the vegetable mixture on six slices. Cover with the remaining slices and grill for 10 minutes. Turn over and grill again for 5 minutes. Serve hot.

Mint Kebab

Makes 8

Ingredients

10g/¼oz mint leaves, finely chopped

500g/1lb 2oz goat's cheese, drained

2 tsp cornflour

10 cashew nuts, roughly chopped

½ tsp ground black pepper

1 tsp amchoor*

Salt to taste

Refined vegetable oil for frying

Method

- Mix together all the ingredients, except the oil. Knead into a soft but firm dough. Divide into 8 lemon-sized balls and flatten them.
- Heat the oil in a saucepan. Deep fry the kebabs on a medium heat till golden brown.
- Serve hot with mint chutney

Vegetable Sevia Upma

(Vegetable Vermicelli Snack)

Serves 4

Ingredients

5 tbsp refined vegetable oil

1 large green pepper, finely chopped

¼ tsp mustard seeds

2 green chillies, slit lengthways

200g/7oz vermicelli

8 curry leaves

Salt to taste

Pinch of asafoetida

50g/1¾oz French beans, finely chopped

1 carrot, finely chopped

50g/1¾oz frozen peas

1 large onion, finely chopped

25g/scant 1oz coriander leaves, finely chopped

Juice of 1 lemon (optional)

Method

- Heat 2 tbsp oil in a saucepan. Fry the green pepper for 2-3 minutes. Set aside.
- Heat 2 tbsp oil in another saucepan. Add the mustard seeds. Let them splutter for 15 seconds.
- Add the green chillies and the vermicelli. Fry for 1-2 minutes on a medium heat, stirring occasionally. Add the curry leaves, salt and asafoetida.
- Sprinkle with a little water and add the fried green pepper, French beans, carrot, peas and onion. Mix well and cook for 3-4 minutes on a medium heat.
- Cover with a lid and cook for another minute.
- Sprinkle the coriander leaves and the lemon juice on top. Serve hot with coconut chutney

Bhel

(Puffed Rice Snack)

Serves 4-6

Ingredients

2 large potatoes, boiled and diced

2 large onions, finely chopped

125g/4½oz roasted peanuts

2 tbsp ground cumin, dry roasted

300g/10oz Bhel Mix

250g/9oz hot and sweet mango chutney

60g/2oz mint chutney

Salt to taste

25g/scant 1oz coriander leaves, chopped

Method

- Mix the potatoes, onions, peanuts and ground cumin with the Bhel Mix. Add both the chutneys and salt. Toss to mix.
- Top with the coriander leaves. Serve immediately.

Sabudana Khichdi

(Sago Snack with Potato and Peanuts)

Serves 6

Ingredients

300g/10oz sago

250ml/8fl oz water

250g/9oz peanuts, coarsely ground

Salt to taste

2 tsp caster sugar

25g/scant 1oz coriander leaves, chopped

2 tbsp refined vegetable oil

1 tsp cumin seeds

5-6 green chillies, finely chopped

100g/3½oz potatoes, boiled and chopped

Method

- Soak the sago overnight in the water. Add the peanuts, salt, caster sugar and coriander leaves and mix well. Set aside.
- Heat the oil in a saucepan. Add the cumin seeds and green chillies. Fry for about 30 seconds.
- Add the potatoes and fry for 1-2 minutes on a medium heat.
- Add the sago mix. Stir and mix well.
- Cover with a lid and cook on a low heat for 2-3 minutes. Serve hot.

Simple Dhokla

(Simple Steamed Cake)

Makes 25

Ingredients

250g/9oz chana dhal*, soaked overnight and drained

2 green chillies

1 tsp ginger paste

Pinch of asafoetida

½ tsp bicarbonate of soda

Salt to taste

2 tbsp refined vegetable oil

½ tsp mustard seeds

4-5 curry leaves

4 tbsp fresh coconut, grated

10g/¼oz coriander leaves, chopped

Method

- Grind the dhal to a coarse paste. Allow to ferment for 6-8 hours.
- Add the green chillies, ginger paste, asafoetida, bicarbonate of soda, salt, 1 tbsp of the oil and a little water. Mix well.
- Grease a 20cm/8in round cake tin and fill it with the batter.
- Steam for 10-12 minutes. Set aside.
- Heat the remaining oil in a saucepan. Add the mustard seeds and curry leaves. Let them splutter for 15 seconds.
- Pour this over the dhoklas. Garnish with the coconut and coriander leaves. Cut into pieces and serve hot.

Jaldi Potato

Serves 4

Ingredients

2 tsp refined vegetable oil

1 tsp cumin seeds

1 green chilli, chopped

½ tsp black salt

1 tsp amchoor*

1 tsp ground coriander

4 large potatoes, boiled and diced

2 tbsp coriander leaves, chopped

Method

- Heat the oil in a saucepan. Add the cumin seeds and let them splutter for 15 seconds.
- Add all the remaining ingredients. Mix well. Cook on a low heat for 3-4 minutes. Serve hot.

Orange Dhokla

(Orange Steamed Cake)

Makes 25

Ingredients

50g/1¾oz semolina

250g/9oz besan*

250ml/8fl oz sour cream

Salt to taste

100ml/3½fl oz water

4 garlic cloves

1cm/½in root ginger

3-4 green chillies

100g/3½oz carrots, grated

¾ tsp bicarbonate of soda

¼ tsp turmeric

Refined vegetable oil for greasing

1 tsp mustard seeds

10-12 curry leaves

50g/1¾oz grated coconut

25g/scant 1oz coriander leaves, finely chopped

Method

- Mix together the semolina, besan, sour cream, salt and water. Set aside to ferment overnight.
- Grind the garlic, ginger and chillies together.
- Add to the fermented batter along with the carrot, bicarbonate of soda and turmeric. Mix well.
- Grease a 20cm/8in round cake tin with a little oil. Pour the batter in it. Steamfor about 20 minutes. Cool and chop into pieces.
- Heat some oil in a saucepan. Add the mustard seeds and curry leaves. Fry them for 30 seconds. Pour this over the dhokla pieces.
- Garnish with the coconut and coriander leaves. Serve hot.

Cabbage Muthia

(Steamed Cabbage Nuggets)

Serves 4

Ingredients

250g/9oz wholemeal flour

100g/3½oz shredded cabbage

½ tsp ginger paste

½ tsp garlic paste

Salt to taste

2 tsp sugar

1 tbsp lemon juice

2 tbsp refined vegetable oil

1 tsp mustard seeds

1 tbsp coriander leaves, chopped

Method

- Mix the flour, cabbage, ginger paste, garlic paste, salt, sugar, lemon juice and 1 tbsp oil. Knead into a pliable dough.
- Make 2 long rolls with the dough. Steam for 15 minutes. Cool and cut into slices. Set aside.
- Heat the remaining oil in a saucepan. Add the mustard seeds. Let them splutter for 15 seconds.
- Add the sliced rolls and fry on a medium heat till brown. Garnish with the coriander leaves and serve hot.

Rava Dhokla

(Steamed Semolina Cake)

Makes 15-18

Ingredients

200g/7oz semolina

240ml/8fl oz sour cream

2 tsp green chillies

Salt to taste

1 tsp red chilli powder

1 tsp ground black pepper

Method

- Mix the semolina and sour cream together. Ferment for 5-6 hours.
- Add the green chillies and salt. Mix well.
- Place the semolina mixture in a 20cm/8in round cake tin. Sprinkle with the chilli powder and pepper. Steam for 10 minutes.
- Cut into pieces and serve hot with mint chutney

Chapatti Upma

(Quick Chapatti Snack)

Serves 4

Ingredients

6 left-over chapattis broken into small bits

2 tbsp refined vegetable oil

¼ tsp mustard seeds

10-12 curry leaves

1 medium-sized onion, chopped

2-3 green chillies, finely chopped

¼ tsp turmeric

Juice of 1 lemon

1 tsp sugar

Salt to taste

10g/¼oz coriander leaves, chopped

Method

- Heat the oil in a saucepan. Add the mustard seeds. Let them splutter for 15 seconds.
- Add the curry leaves, onion, chillies and turmeric. Sauté on a medium heat till the onion turns light brown. Add the chapattis.
- Sprinkle the lemon juice, sugar and salt. Mix well and cook on a medium heat for 5 minutes. Garnish with the coriander leaves and serve hot.

Mung Dhokla

(Steamed Mung Cake)

Makes about 20

Ingredients

250g/9oz mung dhal*, soaked for 2 hours

150ml/5fl oz sour cream

2 tbsp water

Salt to taste

2 grated carrots or 25g/scant 1oz grated cabbage

Method

- Drain the dhal and grind it.
- Add the sour cream and water and ferment for 6 hours. Add the salt and mix well to make the batter.
- Grease a 20cm/8in round cake tin and pour the batter in it. Sprinkle with the carrots or cabbage. Steam for 7-10 minutes.
- Cut into pieces and serve with mint chutney

Mughlai Meat Cutlet

(Rich Meat Cutlet)

Makes 12

Ingredients

1 tsp ginger paste

1 tsp garlic paste

Salt to taste

500g/1lb 2oz boneless lamb, chopped

240ml/8fl oz water

1 tbsp ground cumin

¼ tsp turmeric

Refined vegetable oil for frying

2 eggs, whisked

50g/1¾oz breadcrumbs

Method

- Mix the ginger paste, garlic paste and salt. Marinate the lamb with this mixture for 2 hours.
- In a saucepan, cook the lamb with the water on a medium heat till tender. Reserve the stock and set the lamb aside.
- Add the cumin and turmeric to the stock. Mix well.
- Transfer the stock to a saucepan and simmer till the water evaporates. Marinate the lamb again with this mixture for 30 minutes.
- Heat the oil in a saucepan. Dip each lamb piece in the whisked egg, roll in the breadcrumbs and fry till light brown. Serve hot.

Masala Vada

(Spicy Fried Dumpling)

Makes 15

Ingredients

300g/10oz chana dhal*, soaked in 500ml/16fl oz water for 3-4 hours

50g/1¾oz onion, finely chopped

25g/scant 1oz coriander leaves, chopped

25g/scant 1oz dill leaves, finely chopped

½ tsp cumin seeds

Salt to taste

3 tbsp refined vegetable oil plus extra for deep frying

Method

- Coarsely grind the dhal. Mix with all the ingredients, except the oil.
- Add 3 tbsp of oil to the dhal mixture. Make round, flat patties.
- Heat the remaining oil in a frying pan. Deep fry the patties. Serve hot.

Cabbage Chivda

(Cabbage and Beaten Rice Snack)

Serves 4

Ingredients

100g/3½oz cabbage, finely chopped

Salt to taste

3 tbsp refined vegetable oil

125g/4½oz peanuts

150g/5½oz chana dhal*, roasted

1 tsp mustard seeds

Pinch of asafoetida

200g/7oz poha*, soaked in water

1 tsp ginger paste

4 tsp sugar

1½ tbsp lemon juice

25g/scant 1oz coriander leaves, chopped

Method

- Mix the cabbage with the salt and set aside for 10 minutes.
- Heat 1 tbsp oil in a frying pan. Fry the peanuts and chana dhal for 2 minutes on a medium heat. Drain and set aside.
- Heat the remaining oil in a frying pan. Fry the mustard seeds, asafoetida and cabbage for 2 minutes. Sprinkle a little water, cover with a lid and cook on a low heat for 5 minutes. Add the poha, ginger paste, sugar, lemon juice and salt. Mix well and cook for 10 minutes.
- Garnish with the coriander leaves, fried peanuts and dhal. Serve hot.

Bread Besan Bhajji

(Bread and Gram Flour Snack)

Makes 32

Ingredients

175g/6oz besan*

1250ml/5fl oz water

½ tsp ajowan seeds

Salt to taste

Refined vegetable oil for deep frying

8 bread slices, halved

Method

- Make a thick batter by mixing the besan with the water. Add the ajowan seeds and salt. Whisk well.
- Heat the oil in a frying pan. Dip the bread pieces in the batter and fry till golden brown. Serve hot.

Methi Seekh Kebab

(Skewered Mint Kebab with Fenugreek Leaves)

Makes 8-10

Ingredients

100g/3½oz fenugreek leaves, chopped

3 large potatoes, boiled and mashed

1 tsp ginger paste

1 tsp garlic paste

4 green chillies, finely chopped

1 tsp ground cumin

1 tsp ground coriander

½ tsp garam masala

Salt to taste

2 tbsp breadcrumbs

Refined vegetable oil for basting

Method

- Mix together all the ingredients, except the oil. Shape into patties.
- Skewer and cook on a charcoal grill, basting with the oil and turning occasionally. Serve hot.

Jhinga Hariyali

(Green Prawn)

Makes 20

Ingredients

Salt to taste

Juice of 1 lemon

20 prawns, shelled and de-veined (retain the tail)

75g/2½oz mint leaves, finely chopped

75g/2½oz coriander leaves, chopped

1 tsp ginger paste

1 tsp garlic paste

Pinch of garam masala

1 tbsp refined vegetable oil

1 small onion, sliced

Method

- Rub salt and lemon juice on the prawns. Set aside for 20 minutes.
- Grind together 50g/1¾oz mint leaves, 50g/1¾oz coriander leaves, ginger paste, garlic paste and the garam masala.
- Add to the prawns and set aside for 30 minutes. Sprinkle the oil on top.
- Skewer the prawns and cook on a charcoal grill, turning occasionally.
- Garnish with the remaining coriander and mint leaves, and the sliced onion. Serve hot.

Methi Adai

(Fenugreek Crêpe)

Makes 20-22

Ingredients

100g/3½oz rice

100g/3½oz urad dhal*

100g/3½oz mung dhal*

100g/3½oz chana dhal*

100g/3½oz masoor dhal*

Pinch of asafoetida

6-7 curry leaves

Salt to taste

50g/1¾oz fresh fenugreek leaves, chopped

Refined vegetable oil for greasing

Method

- Soak the rice and dhals together for 3-4 hours.
- Drain the rice and dhal and add the asafoetida, curry leaves and the salt to them. Grind coarsely and set aside to ferment for 7 hours. Add the fenugreek leaves.
- Grease a frying pan and heat it. Add a tbsp of the fermented mixture and spread to form a pancake. Pour some oil around the edges and cook on a medium heat for 3-4 minutes. Flip and cook for 2 more minutes.
- Repeat for the rest of the batter. Serve hot with coconut chutney

Peas Chaat

Serves 4

Ingredients

2 tsp refined vegetable oil

½ tsp cumin seeds

300g/10oz canned green peas

½ tsp amchoor*

¼ tsp turmeric

¼ tsp garam masala

1 tsp lemon juice

5cm/2in root ginger, peeled and julienned

Method

- Heat the oil in a saucepan. Add the cumin seeds and let them splutter for 15 seconds. Add the peas, amchoor, turmeric and garam masala. Mix well and cook for 2-3 minutes, stirring occasionally.
- Garnish with the lemon juice and the ginger. Serve hot.

Shingada

(Bengali Savoury)

Makes 8-10

Ingredients

2 tbsp refined vegetable oil plus extra for deep frying

1 tsp cumin seeds

200g/7oz boiled peas

2 potatoes, boiled and chopped

1 tsp ground coriander

Salt to taste

For the pastry:

350g/12oz plain white flour

¼ tsp salt

A little water

Method

- Heat 2 tbsp oil in a saucepan. Add the cumin seeds. Let them splutter for 15 seconds. Add the peas, potatoes, ground coriander and salt. Mix well and fry on a medium heat for 5 minutes. Set aside.
- Make dough cones with the pastry ingredients, like in the Potato Samosa recipe. Fill the cones with the vegetable mixture and seal.
- Heat the remaining oil in a frying pan. Deep fry the cones on a medium heat till golden brown. Serve hot with mint chutney

Onion Bhajia

(Onion Fritters)

Makes 20

Ingredients

250g/9oz besan*

4 large onions, thinly sliced

Salt to taste

½ tsp turmeric

150ml/5fl oz water

Refined vegetable oil for frying

Method

- Mix the besan, onions, salt and turmeric together. Add the water and mix well.
- Heat the oil in a frying pan. Add spoonfuls of the mixture and deep fry till golden. Drain on absorbent paper and serve hot.

Bagani Murgh

(Chicken in Cashew Paste)

Makes 12

Ingredients

500g/1lb 2oz boneless chicken, diced

1 small onion, sliced

1 tomato, sliced

1 cucumber, sliced

1 tsp ginger paste

1 tsp garlic paste

2 green chillies, finely chopped

10g/¼oz mint leaves, ground

10g/¼oz coriander leaves, ground

Salt to taste

For the marinade:

6-7 cashew nuts, ground to a paste

2 tbsp single cream

Method

- Mix the marinade ingredients together. Marinate the chicken with this mixture for 4-5 hours.
- Skewer and cook on a charcoal grill, turning occasionally.
- Garnish with the onion, tomato and cucumber. Serve hot.

Potato Tikki

(Potato Patties)

Makes 12

Ingredients

4 large potatoes, boiled and mashed

1 tsp ginger paste

1 tsp garlic paste

Juice of 1 lemon

1 large onion, finely chopped

25g/scant 1oz coriander leaves, chopped

¼ tsp chilli powder

Salt to taste

2 tbsp rice flour

3 tbsp refined vegetable oil

Method

- Mix the potatoes with the ginger paste, garlic paste, lemon juice, onion, coriander leaves, chilli powder and salt. Knead well. Shape into patties.
- Dust the patties with rice flour.
- Heat the oil in a frying pan. Shallow fry the patties on a medium heat till golden brown. Drain and serve hot with mint chutney.

Batata Vada

(Batter Fried Potato Dumpling)

Makes 12-14

Ingredients

1 tsp refined vegetable oil plus extra for deep frying

½ tsp mustard seeds

½ tsp urad dhal*

½ tsp turmeric

5 potatoes, boiled and mashed

Salt to taste

Juice of 1 lemon

250g/9oz besan*

Pinch of asafoetida

120ml/4fl oz water

Method

- Heat 1 tsp oil in a frying pan. Add the mustard seeds, urad dhal and turmeric. Let them splutter for 15 seconds.
- Pour this over the potatoes. Also add salt and lemon juice. Mix well.
- Divide the potato mixture into walnut-sized balls. Set aside.
- Mix the besan, asafoetida, salt and water to make the batter.
- Heat the remaining oil in a frying pan. Dip the potato balls in the batter and deep fry till golden. Drain and serve with mint chutney.

Mini Chicken Kebab

Makes 8

Ingredients

350g/12oz chicken, minced

125g/4½oz besan*

1 large onion, finely chopped

½ tsp ginger paste

½ tsp garlic paste

1 tsp lemon juice

¼ tsp green cardamom powder

1 tbsp coriander leaves, chopped

Salt to taste

1 tbsp sesame seeds

Method

- Mix together all the ingredients, except the sesame seeds.
- Divide the mixture into small balls and sprinkle with sesame seeds.
- Bake in an oven at 190ºC (375ºF, Gas Mark 5) for 25 minutes. Serve hot with mint chutney.

Lentil Rissole

Makes 12

Ingredients

2 tbsp refined vegetable oil plus extra for shallow frying

2 small onions, finely chopped

2 carrots, finely chopped

600g/1lb 5oz masoor dhal*

500ml/16fl oz water

2 tbsp ground coriander

Salt to taste

25g/scant 1oz coriander leaves, chopped

100g/3½oz breadcrumbs

2 tbsp plain white flour

1 egg, whisked

Method

- Heat 1 tbsp oil in a frying pan. Add the onions and carrots and fry on a medium heat for 2-3 minutes, stirring frequently. Add the masoor dhal, water, ground coriander and salt. Simmer for 30 minutes, stirring.
- Add the coriander leaves and half the breadcrumbs. Mix well.
- Mould into sausage shapes and coat with the flour. Dip the rissoles in the whisked egg and roll in the remaining breadcrumbs. Set aside.
- Heat the remaining oil. Shallow fry the rissoles till golden, flipping once. Serve hot with green coconut chutney.

Nutritious Poha

Serves 4

Ingredients

1 tbsp refined vegetable oil

125g/4½oz peanuts

1 onion, finely chopped

¼ tsp turmeric

Salt to taste

1 potato, boiled and chopped

200g/7oz poha*, soaked for 5 minutes and drained

1 tsp lemon juice

1 tbsp coriander leaves, chopped

Method

- Heat the oil in a saucepan. Fry the peanuts, onion, turmeric and salt on a medium heat for 2-3 minutes.
- Add the potato and poha. Stir-fry on a low heat till evenly mixed.
- Garnish with the lemon juice and coriander leaves. Serve hot.

Beans Usal

(Beans in Spicy Gravy)

Serves 4

Ingredients

300g/10oz masoor dhal*, soaked in hot water for 20 minutes

¼ tsp turmeric

Salt to taste

50g/1¾oz French beans, finely chopped

240ml/8fl oz water

1 tbsp refined vegetable oil

¼ tsp mustard seeds

A few curry leaves

Salt to taste

Method

- Mix the dhal, turmeric and salt together. Grind to a coarse paste.
- Steam for 20-25 minutes. Set aside to cool for 20 minutes. Crumble the mixture with your fingers. Set aside.
- Cook the French beans with the water and a little salt in a saucepan on a medium heat till soft. Set aside.
- Heat the oil in a saucepan. Add the mustard seeds. Let them splutter for 15 seconds. Add the curry leaves and the crumbled dhal.
- Stir-fry for about 3-4 minutes on a medium heat till soft. Add the cooked beans and mix well. Serve hot.

Bread Chutney Pakoda

Serves 4

Ingredients

250g/9oz besan*

150ml/5fl oz water

½ tsp ajowan seeds

125g/4½oz mint chutney

12 slices of bread

Refined vegetable oil for deep frying

Method

- Mix the besan with the water to make a batter of a pancake-mix consistency. Add the ajowan seeds and whisk lightly. Set aside.
- Spread the mint chutney on a bread slice and place another on top. Repeat for all the bread slices. Cut them diagonally into half.
- Heat the oil in a frying pan. Dip the sandwiches in the batter and fry on a medium heat till golden brown. Serve hot with ketchup.

Methi Khakra Delight

(Fenugreek Snack)

Makes 16

Ingredients

50g/1¾oz fresh fenugreek leaves, finely chopped

300g/10oz wholemeal flour

1 tsp chilli powder

¼ tsp turmeric

½ tsp ground coriander

1 tbsp refined vegetable oil

Salt to taste

120ml/4fl oz water

Method

- Mix all the ingredients together. Knead into a soft but firm dough.
- Divide the dough into 16 lemon-sized balls. Roll out into very thin discs.
- Heat a flat pan. Place the discs on the flat pan and cook till crisp. Repeat for the other side. Store in an airtight container.

Green Cutlet

Makes 12

Ingredients

200g/7oz spinach, finely chopped

4 potatoes, boiled and mashed

200g/7oz mung dhal*, boiled and mashed

25g/scant 1oz coriander leaves, chopped

2 green chillies, finely chopped

1 tsp garam masala

1 large onion, finely chopped

Salt to taste

1 tsp garlic paste

1 tsp ginger paste

Refined vegetable oil for frying

250g/9oz breadcrumbs

Method

- Mix the spinach and potatoes together. Add the mung dhal, coriander leaves, green chillies, garam masala, onion, salt, garlic paste and ginger paste. Knead well.
- Divide the mixture into walnut-sized portions and shape each into cutlets.
- Heat the oil in a frying pan. Roll the cutlets in the breadcrumbs and shallow fry till golden brown. Serve hot.

Handvo

(Savoury Semolina Cake)

Serves 4

Ingredients

100g/3½oz semolina

125g/4½oz besan*

200g/7oz yoghurt

25g/scant 1oz bottle gourd, grated

1 carrot, grated

25g/scant 1oz green peas

½ tsp turmeric

½ tsp chilli powder

½ tsp ginger paste

½ tsp garlic paste

1 green chilli, finely chopped

Salt to taste

Pinch of asafoetida

½ tsp bicarbonate of soda

4 tbsp refined vegetable oil

¾ tsp mustard seeds

½ tsp sesame seeds

Method

- Mix the semolina, besan and yoghurt in a saucepan. Add the grated bottle gourd and carrot and the peas.
- Add the turmeric, chilli powder, ginger paste, garlic paste, green chilli, salt and asafoetida to make the batter. It should have the consistency of a cake batter. If not, add a few tablespoons of water.
- Add the bicarbonate of soda and stir well. Set aside.
- Heat the oil in a saucepan. Add the mustard and sesame seeds. Let them splutter for 15 seconds.
- Pour the batter in the saucepan. Cover with a lid and cook on a low heat for 10-12 minutes.
- Uncover and flip the set batter carefully, using a spatula. Cover again and cook on a low heat for 15 more minutes.
- Pierce with a fork to check if done. If cooked, the fork will come out clean. Serve hot.

Ghugra

(Crescents with Savoury Vegetable Centres)

Serves 4

Ingredients

5 tbsp refined vegetable oil plus extra for deep frying

Pinch of asafoetida

400g/14oz canned peas, ground

250ml/8fl oz water

Salt to taste

5cm/2in root ginger, finely chopped

2 tsp lemon juice

1 tbsp coriander leaves, chopped

350g/12oz wholemeal flour

Method

- Heat 2 tbsp oil in a saucepan. Add the asafoetida. When it splutters, add the peas and 120ml/4fl oz water. Cook on a medium heat for 3 minutes.

- Add the salt, ginger and lemon juice. Mix well and cook for another 5 minutes. Sprinkle the coriander leaves on top and set aside.

- Knead the flour with the salt, remaining water and 3 tbsp oil. Divide into small balls and roll out into round discs of 10cm/4in diameter.

- Place some pea mixture on each disc so that half the disc is covered with the mixture. Fold the other half over to make a 'D' shape. Seal by pressing the edges together.

- Heat the oil. Fry the ghugras on a medium heat till golden. Serve hot.

Banana Kebab

Makes 20

Ingredients

6 green bananas

1 tsp ginger paste

250g/9oz besan*

25g/scant 1oz coriander leaves, chopped

½ tsp chilli powder

1 tsp amchoor*

Juice of 1 lemon

Salt to taste

240ml/8fl oz refined vegetable oil for shallow frying

Method

- Boil the bananas in their skins for 10-15 minutes. Drain and peel.

- Mix with the remaining ingredients, except the oil. Shape into patties.

- Heat the oil in a frying pan. Shallow fry the patties till golden. Serve hot.

Lightning Source UK Ltd.
Milton Keynes UK
UKHW021856220421
382471UK00003B/248